HEART FAILURE

THINGS YOU SHOULD KNOW
(QUESTIONS AND ANSWERS)

By Rumi Michael Leigh

Introduction

I would like to thank and congratulate you for purchasing this book, " *Heart Failure, things you should know (questions and answers)*" series.

This book will help you understand, revise and have a good general knowledge and keywords of heart failure and how it affects the lives of people with this disease.

Thanks again for purchasing this book, I hope you enjoy it !

Chapter 1

1) What is heart failure?

- This is when the heart is too weak to effectively pump blood to the organs.

2) What is the function of the heart?

- Its function is to supply and pump blood to the organs of the body.

3) Do the right and left side of the heart have the same function?

- No.

4) What is the function of the right side of the heart?

- The supply of oxygen to the lungs.

5) What is the function of the left side of the heart?

- The supply of oxygen to the body.

6) How many types of heart failure are there?

- There are two types of heart failure.

7) What are the types of heart failure?

- Right-sided and left-sided heart failure.

8) What type of heart failure is the most common?

- Left-sided heart failure.

9) Can you have a left and right-sided heart failure at the same time?

- Yes.

10) Does heart failure mean that the heart has stopped working?

- No.

Chapter 2

1) Can children also have heart failure?

- Yes, also in newborns, teenagers, etc.

2) What is hypertension?

- It is a medical condition whereby the blood pressure is too high.

3) Can hypertension lead to heart failure?

- Yes.

4) Can alcohol abuse lead to heart failure?

- Yes.

5) Can cocaine abuse lead to heart failure?

- Yes.

6) Why do sportsmen/sportswomen have lower heart rates?

- They have lower heart rates because their heart pumps enough blood to the body with each contraction.

7) Is chest pain always of cardiac origin?

- No.

8) What can relieve chest pain associated with angina pectoris?

-   Rest and medications.

9) What is systolic?

-   This is when the heart contracts.

10) What is diastolic?

-   This is when the heart relaxes.

Chapter 3

1) What is left-sided heart failure?

- This is when the ventricle is rigid, thus does not contract sufficiently. This makes the blood flow back to the lungs through the atrium and thereby causing pulmonary symptoms.

2) What is right-sided heart failure?

- This is when the ventricles do not pump out blood sufficiently, thus blood flows back into the vena cava that can eventually cause weight gain, peripheral edema, etc.

3) What is ejection fraction?

- This is the percentage of blood that is pumped out by the left ventricle with each heartbeat.

4) What is considered a normal ejection fraction?

- An ejection fraction between 50% and 70%.

5) What is considered a low ejection fraction?

- An ejection fraction lesser than 50%.

6) What is considered a very low ejection fraction?

-      An ejection fraction lesser than 40%.

7)   Does a normal ejection fraction indicate the absence of heart failure?

-      No, you can have a normal ejection fraction and still have heart failure.

8)   What is considered as a high ejection fraction?

-      An ejection fraction higher than 75%.

9)   What can cause heart murmurs?

-      The narrowing of the heart valves.

10) What is claudification?

-      It is pain in a lower limb when walking.

Chapter 4

1) What is a coronary heart disease?

- It is a decrease in blood flow to the heart due to the narrowing of the coronary arteries by fatty plaques.

2) What can cause fatty plaques developed around the coronary arteries?

- Atherosclerosis.

3) Name the factors of coronary heart disease.

- Obesity, overweight, smoking, diabetes, sedentary lifestyle, etc.

4) What is collateral circulation of the heart?

- Collateral circulation consists of small blood vessels that redirect blood around a blocked artery.

5) Name a common sign or symptom of coronary heart disease.

- Chest pain due to physical activities that may be relieved with rest or without rest.

6) How can coronary heart disease be diagnosed?

- Coronary heart disease can be diagnosed by blood test, electrocardiogram, stress test, etc.

7) What is arterectomy?

- This is the removal of plaque from the artery through surgical procedures.

8) What is cardiac decompensation?

- This is when the signs and symptoms of heart failure get worse.

9) Name 3 systems of cardiac decompensation.

- Ischemic disorder, the renin-angiotensin system and cardiac remodeling.

10) What is an ischemic disorder?

- This is when there is an insufficient blood supply to the tissues of the body.

Chapter 5

1) What is cardiac remodeling?

- This is the change in shape, structure, size and function of the heart.

2) Give another name of cardiac remodeling.

- Ventricular remodeling.

3) What is the main cause of cardiac remodeling?

- Cardiac dysfunction.

4) What is arrhythmia?

- This is an irregular heart rhythm. It is when the heart beats too fast or too slow.

5) What is another name given to arrhythmia?

- It can also be called dysrhythmia.

6) What is bradycardia?

- This is slow heartbeat.

7) What is tachycardia?

- This is fast heartbeat.

8) What is the normal heart rate?

- The normal heart rate is between 60 to 100 beats per minute.

9) What is anemia?

- This is an insufficient red blood cell count.

10) Can anemia lead to heart failure?

- Yes.

Chapter 6

1) What is edema?

- Characterized by swelling, edema is the accumulation of fluid in the body's tissues.

2) In what part of the body is there congestion if there is right-sided heart failure?

- At the lower limbs with edema.

3) What is the use of diuretics in cardiac insufficiency?

- Diuretics are used for the treatment of edema.

4) What is the cause of edema in the arm?

- It could be due to a venous obstruction or breast surgery.

5) Is edema in the lower limb an origin of the right or left-sided heart failure?

- Right-sided heart failure.

6) Can edema migrate?

- Yes.

7) What is the normal capillary refill time?

- Less than 2 seconds.

8) What can cause varicose veins?

-   Varicose veins can be caused by defective vein valves.

9) What can cause thick finger nails and slow their growth?

-   Arterial insufficiency.

10) What can cause flat jugular veins?

-   Hypovolemia and dehydration.

Chapter 7

1) What are the medications for heart failure?

- Beta blockers, anticoagulants, diuretics, etc.

2) What is the function of the conversion enzyme inhibitor?

- It is used for the treatment of heart failure. It prevents the vasoconstriction effect.

3) What is the function of a beta-blocker?

- It reduces the work of the heart; thus, it slows down the heart.

4) A beta-blocker acts on which system of the heart; the sympathetic or parasympathetic?

- The sympathetic system.

5) What is hyperkalemia?

- Hyperkalemia is a high potassium level in the blood.

6) What are some of the risk factors of hyperkalemia?

- Congestive heart failure, HIV, diabetes, etc.

7) What is the function of potassium in the heart?

\-   Potassium enables proper contraction of the heart; thus, it enables the heart to pump blood efficiently.

8) What part of the body regulates potassium?

\-   The kidneys.

9) What is the danger of diuretics in heart failure?

\-   Certain diuretics make you get rid of potassium through urine.

10) What is cardiomyopathy?

\-   It is a disease of the heart muscle.

Chapter 8

1) What are the factors of risk of myocardial infarction also known as a heart attack?

- A poor diet, age, a lack of physical activity, atherosclerosis, diabetes, heredity, etc.

2) Does rest relieve chest pain from myocardial infarction?

- No.

3) What are the characteristics of scar tissues of the myocardium?

- Scar tissues are rigid and do not have the same power of contraction.

4) What is diaphoresis?

- This is an unusual excessive sweating.

5) Is diaphoresis the origin of right or left-sided heart failure?

- A left-sided heart failure.

6) What is sleep apnea?

- Sleep apnea is a sleep disorder when breathing stops for a brief period.

7) Can sleep apnea cause heart failure?

-    Yes.

8) How can sleep apnea cause heart failure?

-    It causes severe fatigue.

9) What is a pacemaker?

-    It is a device that helps the heart against arrhythmias.

10) In a situation where the heartbeat is too slow, what is normally done in order to maintain a normal heartbeat?

-    An implant of a pacemaker.

Chapter 9

1) In a situation where the heartbeat is too fast, what is normally done in order to maintain a normal heartbeat?

- Medications, radiofrequency ablation.

2) What is hyperthyroidism?

- This is an over secretion of thyroxine hormone which can abnormally accelerate the body's metabolism.

3) Can hyperthyroidism lead to heart failure?

- Yes.

4) How could hyperthyroidism lead to heart failure?

- Hyperthyroidism makes the heart work at a faster pace than normal which could overwork the heart.

5) Is a decrease in blood pressure a cause of left or right-sided heart failure?

- Left-sided heart failure.

6) Are crackling rattles a cause of left or right-sided heart failure?

- Right-sided heart failure.

7) What is hepatomegaly?

-   This is an abnormally enlarged liver size.

8) Is hepatomegaly a cause of left or right-sided heart failure?

-   Right-sided heart failure.

9) What is dyspnea?

-   This is difficulty in breathing.

10) Is dyspnea a cause of left or right-sided heart failure?

-   Left-sided heart failure.

Chapter 10

1) What is orthopnea?

- This is difficulty breathing while lying down.

2) Is orthopnea a cause of left or right-sided heart failure?

- Left-sided heart failure.

3) What is cyanosis?

- This is a bluish coloration of the skin or the mucus membranes due to insufficient oxygen supply.

4) Is cyanosis a cause of left or right-sided heart failure?

- Left-sided heart failure.

5) What is asthenia?

- This is weakness, a lack of physical strength in the body.

6) Is asthenia a cause of left or right-sided heart failure?

- Left-sided heart failure.

7) What is ascites?

- It is an abnormal buildup of fluids in the body that can be caused by congestive heart failure, cirrhosis of the liver, etc.

8) Is ascites a cause of left or right-sided heart failure?

- Left-sided heart failure.

9) What is nocturia?

- This is the need to frequently urinate at night.

10) Is nocturia a cause of left or right-sided heart failure?

- Right-sided heart failure.

Chapter 11

1) What is the optimal oxygen saturation?

- 100%.

2) Is the decrease in oxygen saturation a cause of left or right-sided heart failure?

- Left-sided heart failure.

3) Is weight increase a cause of left or right-sided heart failure?

- Both left and right-sided heart failure.

4) What is oliguria?

- This is a condition of low urine output.

5) Is oliguria a cause of left or right-sided heart failure?

- Left-sided heart failure.

6) What is anuria?

- This is kidney failure. The kidneys fail to produce urine.

7) Is anuria a cause of left or right-sided heart failure?

- Left-sided heart failure.

8) Is jugular vein turgor a cause of left or right-sided heart failure?

-   Right-sided heart failure.

9) Is tachypnea a cause of left or right-sided heart failure?

-   Left-sided heart failure.

10) Can people with heart failure live normal lives?

-   Yes, if they change their lifestyle and with appropriate treatments and medications and awareness of their condition.

Conclusion

Thank you again for purchasing this book. I hope it has helped you in your journey to understanding heart failure and how it affects the people around you who suffer from this disease.

Thank you.

www.ingramcontent.com/pod-product-compliance
Lightning Source LLC
Chambersburg PA
CBHW051144250726
48655CB00007B/3230